Coach, I didn't run because...
Excuses not to Run

Coach Dean

authorHOUSE®

AuthorHouse™
1663 Liberty Drive, Suite 200
Bloomington, IN 47403
www.authorhouse.com
Phone: 1-800-839-8640

First published by AuthorHouse 12/4/2008

ISBN: 978-1-4389-1602-6 (sc)

Printed in the United States of America
Bloomington, Indiana

This book is printed on acid-free paper.

Table of Contents

If you really don't want to work out

Then don't.

Scream it from the roof tops.

But STOP the excuses.

Nobody wants to hear them.

Sit your ass down and get the TV remote.

Acknowledgments

It is one thing to talk about writing a book it's quite another getting it done. I thank all the runners who have contributed and inspired this book. But, my biggest thanks go to Christina Heinle, who gave invaluable feedback and kept me on track. Thanks to her, we kept excuses at bay and got it done.

Coach, I didn't run because...

From Excuse to Motivation

Let me tell you a bit about the origins of this book and the original "Excuses Not to Workout" list.

The original excuse list was created over many years by running groups I have coached; specifically the High Performance Running Club and RxRunning & Racing Club in Tempe and Mesa, Arizona and Gilbert's Mesquite High School cross-country team. In addition, a number of non-club individuals have contributed to the ever growing list of excuses.

A portion of excuses date much further back to the late 1970s from the high school years of Greg Mason. Greg's list is courtesy of his Peoria Illinois high school coach. These ancient excuses were extracted from the stone tablets they were written on. It's funny to see how little the excuses have changed over the years.

I also want to set the record straight, these excuses come from runners of all abilities. They are novice first-time runners to thirty-plus year veterans; teenagers to retirees; elite nationally ranked to back-of-the-packers. Be clear on this - no one is exempt!

During team meetings with the running groups we would state goals for the upcoming competitive season. In support of our goals we wanted to include some motivational fodder. In that vein, we would have a contest for the most creative, different or remarkable excuse for someone who didn't get a scheduled workout done during the past year. Duplicates were not allowed, but twists on the former excuses were. Some excuses are derived from real incidents, some are quite fantasy; and yet some are real but seem like fantasy. In the end, everyone would vote for the "best" excuse. Of course, prizes and prides were at stake. Everyone wanted to have the best excuse not to get a run in. I do not - in any way – believe this book contains all the excuses for which not to workout. Quite the contrary, I firmly believe that this is a starting point from which everyone can build. There are as many excuses as there are people and these excuses are as unique as the person creating the excuse.

The book elaborates on the five major excuses people use for not working out derived from a landmark survey conducted by The National Sporting Goods Association (NSGA) in 1993. The NSGA did a survey of thousands of inactive people (less than 25 days a year fitness activity) and active people (more than 150 days a year of fitness activity). As you will see, the results were surprising and yet not so surprising.

This book is not just for runners however. Everyone who has ever endeavored to get in shape, embarked on a fitness program or stayed on a diet can benefit from reading this book. Excuses know no boundaries.

Over the 35 plus years of excuses during my own non-running periods, (yes, I've used a good portion of these excuses) and hearing excuses by so many others - I realized it would be handy to create a list to make it easier for everyone to easily choose an excuse. Voila! The handy-dandy every-excuse-you-ever-wanted-to-use excuse list is here. Now, in your running log just enter: Tuesday, #47; Wednesday, #141. It expedites conversations between runners – "It was a #221 day." In reality this is a very practical, efficient long-time needed tool.

The point of this book is to clearly demonstrate that anything can become an excuse - **real or imagined.** Ok, another purpose of this book is simply a catharsis and as a salute to every runner I know.

Get Serious About Excuses

Some idiots over the past 30 years or so... since the running boom of the 1970s... have lead people to believe that working out is some pleasurable, smile producing, euphoric activity. Liars!

Working out is our way to compensate for inactivity in the rest of our Information Age lives. We don't hunt for our food. Most of us don't grow our own food. We don't regularly fend off saber-toothed tigers. We sit at desks. We stare at computers. And we drive through the drive-thru and super-size it. Do you think cavemen went for daily runs on their own? Not without a tiger chasing their ass every step of the way!

So, acknowledge up front that most of the time getting or staying in shape is hard work. And to state the obvious – if it were easy then everyone would do it. If you are starting a new workout regimen it's even harder. Let's admit it, it downright sucks some times. I've had the displeasure of coming back after many injuries and surgeries. It sucks getting back in shape. I would much rather stay in shape than have to regain being in shape!

If you can't cope with the short term fact that working out often sucks and the pay-off is often in STOPPING your workout; and if you cannot see that the long term pay off is just that, long term; you probably have already used most of these excuses.

Don't get me totally wrong. There are days that are just fantastic. Once you are in shape they happen more often. And you only get in shape by avoiding excuses and getting your ass out the door. This is just a reality check – stop thinking it's going to be easy to get in shape. Stop thinking it's going to be pleasurable. Now, get used to getting out and doing it anyway!

Using an excuse is purely a mind game. The trick is to find a way to play the game and not just sit on the bench watching the game. So, what's your mindset? Are you in the game or just watching from the bench (aka couch)? Anyone, anytime, can find an excuse not to do something. Those who have an overriding purpose or reason for doing something will simply not use excuses... they will just do it.

5

Activity Related Excuses

Working out doesn't use more energy. It gives back far more than it takes. The more fit you are the more work you can do. If you want to have the energy to go to the park and play with your kids, get out and run. If you want to have energy to do yard work more effortlessly, get out and run. If you want more energy to play, get out and run. If you want more energy to shop in the malls, get out and run. As your fitness level increases your ability to use oxygen and energy sources becomes more efficient. Everything you do will take comparatively less energy. You'll get that bounce back in your step!

Coach I didn't run because...

1. I swam today.
2. I had a golf game.
3. I did my leg weight workout.
4. You get faster when you don't do back-to-back workout days.
5. I trained too hard yesterday.
6. I have to unpack, clean the pool, clean the cabinets, line the cabinets, organize the closets, rake the front yard, and mow the back yard.
7. I'd rather play soccer.
8. I really will feel better (for everyone else) AFTER the run.
9. If I ride a bike, I'll get done sooner.
10. I was watching Olympics.
11. I had a great run yesterday.
12. I've fallen and I can't get up.
13. I'm tapering for the Summer 5k Series.

14. ..sorry, I'm on the phone right now.

15. I felt undeserving to run because I paid my club dues late.

16. My water bottle fell in the porta-potty.

17. I'm watching my younger siblings.

18. I was passed by a lady with a jog stroller.

19. There wasn't enough time to warm up.

20. I warmed up too much.

21. I haven't trained enough.

22. I didn't have enough sleep.

23. I had too much sleep.

24. I have not had enough weight training.

25. I had too much weight training.

26. I'm building up slowly for next year.

27. I don't want to peak too soon.

28. My girlfriend/boyfriend was unfriendly.

29. My girlfriend/boyfriend was too friendly.

30. He cut me off.

31. I cut him off and thought I was disqualified.

32. I fell down.

33. I'm a "mudder" and it was a too dry.

34. They all jumped but me.

35. I thought they would recall us to the start.

36. I can't run when I'm behind.

37. I can't run when I'm ahead.

38. I can't run.

39. There is too much competition.

40. There is not enough competition.

41. There are too many meets.

42.   There are not enough meets.

43.   Studying comes first.

44.   I never had to run so hard before.

45.   I had to stay home to babysit.

46.   I don't know the pace.

47.   I have to quit to get a job.

48.   I had to clean the kitty litter.

49.   I have to quit to get better grades.

50.   I have homework.

Survey Says…"I Don't Have Enough Time"

The number one complaint of the inactive people was that they lacked sufficient time to work out. I know as a coach of both experienced and novice athletes; I hear the "time" excuse often. I also notice that there are certain individuals who manage to complete workouts in concert with other obligations.

Here is the kicker of the survey: The survey also found that there was virtually no difference in the amount of **actual** free time between the two groups!

Excuse Buster

We all have the same 24 hours in a day and 168 hours per week. Well-to-do individuals cannot buy more and less well-off individuals are not short changed. Neither the intellectually gifted nor the mentally challenged get more. Meticulous detail oriented to-do-listers do not get more time - neither do the fly-by-the-seat-of-your-pants non-planners. Neither methodical plodders nor spastic multi-taskers get more time. And neither 20 year olds nor 52 year olds get more time. So, we have to delve deeper than the objective issue of time available.

I'm an observer of behaviors. One of the things I notice is how much time someone will complain about something; during which they could have already done something about that complaint. I notice skewed perceptions of available time. How is it that 30 minutes is just enough time for some people to squeeze in a workout and others see it as not enough time to barely put on their running shoes?

Dr. Ralph Paffenberger a renowned health researcher (the famous series of Harvard studies) estimates that for every hour of working out you gain two hours of life. This is good news. Well, Ok, if your life sucks then it only means extra time with life sucking. But, most of us might find some comfort and motivation in knowing working out isn't really wasting time but investing in time… with a potential of 100% return on that investment! So, you lost the logic argument – now get your ass out there!

Apparel Related Excuses

What do you "need" to do your run? Do you have to search for everything before you head out to the gym or onto the roads or trails? If you are supposed to run in the morning, put everything out the night before. Wear your running shorts to bed if you have to. Place your socks in your shoes. If you run right after work, pack your bag and place it in your vehicle the night before. You won't zoom out the next morning with coffee in hand and have the excuse of "I forgot my running gear."

For anyone who tends to be a bit scatter-brained (or just working on early senility like me), I strongly recommend that you put your "running essentials" list on a three-by-five card. Use it just like a pilot doing a pre-flight check. Follow your list. Don't jump around on your list. You will inevitably forget to come back to a previous item. Keep the card in your workout bag. The idea is to remove excuses – especially these very preventable ones!

The fact is there are more clothing options today than there ever was. But when it comes down to it, you only needs running shoes, socks, shorts and a shirt (or not) and it doesn't matter what the material is. So get over it. It doesn't matter that your colors match or that they are all matching Puma, Adidas or Nike.

Coach, I didn't run because...

51.   My shoes are too tight.

52.   My shoes are too loose.

53.   My shoes are too old.

54.   My shoes are too new.

55.   My shoes are too light.

56.   My shoes are too heavy.

57. My shoes are the wrong color.

58. My shoes are still attached to my bike.

59. These aren't my shoes.

60. I only have my wife's shoes to run in.

61. My dog ate my shorts.

62. I locked my keys in my shoes.

63. Because I bought my shoes from brand "X" store.

64. I had a flat on my left shoe.

65. My dog chewed up my running hat.

66. I wore high heels this weekend.

67. My brother/sister has my running shoes.

68. My dog ate my running shorts and hid my running shoes.

69. My favorite running shoe style was discontinued.

70. There's a leak in my Camelbak.

71. I have a knot in my sneakers.

72. My aqua-belt has a hole in it.

73. I don't have any Adidas (Asics, Nike, New Balance, Puma, Saucony, Brooks – insert your favorite brand).

74. I forgot my shoes.

75. My favorite shorts are in the wash.

76. My running skirt spankies keep riding up.

77. I don't have any clean running clothes.

78. I don't have my running clothes with me.

Survey Says..."I Don't Have Enough Energy"

Working out more often results and is reported by people to give you more energy not the reverse. You want energy? Get your ass up and workout! Fatigue is not a real thing. It is predominantly a mental thing. There is now ample research supporting the fact that our brains interpret the sensations of our body. Some people interpret sensations as "pain" while others view the same stimulus as "discomfort." At the end of the day some interpret their sensations as "wiped out" and can't do anything but grab the remote control and a beer while others interpret it as a "call to action" to wake up and get going!

Similarly, deep into a killer workout on the track this mental aspect of fatigue is nicely demonstrated. On the tenth of sixteen 400 meter repeats everyone reports being so tired they're not sure they can complete the workout. Get them to refocus on one repetition at a time and they get through them. Here's the real "aha" – when asked to push the last one or two repeats (after the whining is done) what do you think happens? Nine times out of ten, split times are faster than any of the other fourteen repetitions. It is a vivid example of our interpretation of fatigue and the energy we have, or think we don't have. If in fact there was no energy left, you would physically not be able to run those last repeats faster. Yet they did.

Excuse Buster

Inertia is the real issue. This is really a corollary to the energy issue. A body at rest will want to stay at rest. Once you stop and put your feet up - like at the end of a long day - odds are against you getting going again. Keep your ass moving!

If in fact, we were physiologically fatigued to the point we "couldn't do another rep" or "couldn't possibly go faster" then our bodies simply wouldn't respond – regardless of will power and motivation. 100% is 100%. 100% by definition is everything. There is no such thing as giving 110%. The fact is we usually give far less than 100% and that is why we can and do perform more than we thought possible. Period.

The mental construct and interpretation of our sensations are what "told us" we were tired. So, get over it! You aren't as tired as you think. You do have the energy. Now get your ass out there!

Food Related Excuses

Stop taking eating for granted. We are on autopilot too often when it comes to our nutritional needs. Planning is the key.

The evening before, think through your next day. When will you have a break? Will fluids and nutrition be available? Can you avoid fast food? If you work out after work, plan on a snack in mid-afternoon. If you have to, set your computer reminder for your three o'clock healthy snack break. Don't give in to the candy vending machine temptation down the hall. Plan ahead and bring a healthy snack. Pack some easy to carry non-perishable snacks like pretzels, trail mix, low fat cracker, etc. Pack fresh fruit if your daily environment allows. It's not going to be a pretty sight if you pack a banana and it will be outside in 110F degrees. If you're going to be on the road, do an Internet search for restaurants in the area. Do not leave it to chance that you will find a healthy alternative. Or purchase backpacking food that all you need to do is add hot water.

Fill water bottles and have them waiting for you in the refrigerator and grab one on the way out the door in the morning. Ok, that does require that you actually remember to grab them. During the summer months, freeze water bottles to take along with you on your run. The ice will slowly melt during the day providing cool water for hours.

So, avoid excuses and put your brief case (or something else you absolutely have to have with you when you leave… like car keys) in the refrigerator too. This way you will have to visit the fridge in your morning rush out the door.

Stop forcing yourself to eat things you do not like. Visit a Registered Dietician who specializes in athletes and active lifestyles. They will find alternatives with the right nutrition values.

If you are a do-it-yourselfer then my recommendation is that you obtain Nancy Clark's publications. They are the best available. No fads, just facts. Here are some of her publications: Sports Nutrition Guidebook,

The Cyclist's Food Guide, Nancy Clark's Food Guide for Marathoners, and the Home Study course for Sports Nutrition Guidebook.

Coach, I didn't run because...

79. Two words: Chai Tea.
80. I have explosive diarrhea and I'm afraid my shorts will catch on fire.
81. I had a late lunch.
82. I didn't have my coffee today.
83. My body functions/fluids wanted to depart my body!
84. I ate too much.
85. I didn't eat enough.
86. I'm weak from lack of nourishment.
87. I need wheat germ oil.
88. I need yogurt.
89. I need vitamin C.
90. I drank too much soda yesterday.
91. I don't have enough salt in my system.
92. I'm dehydrated.

Survey Says... "I'm Not Motivated to Workout"

Motivation is a very complex construct. But, if working out is not part of your value system you are working against the flow. Your motivation to "just do it" will gravitate towards "just do something else" at the first opportunity. Re-evaluate why you want to work out. There is no rah-rah motivational speech that is going to overpower your basic value system – at least not for long.

Excuse Buster

It comes down to priorities which are established through our values. More specifically if you are one of those people who believe that "everything" is a priority then you will ultimately fail. You scatter your time and energy. You are neither effective nor efficient. Set priorities, not everything is #1. If you do not view working out as something that ultimately enhances your life and pays back more than it takes then you won't work out. It's pretty simple. Working out must be seen as time for yourself; time to "feed" yourself; time to rejuvenate yourself; time to do something just for you not everyone else in your life; time to invest in order to ultimately get back more time.

If these self-serving reasons don't motivate you and instead you are "motivated" by giving everything of yourself to others then the bonus to working out is that you inevitably will have more energy to give to others. In other words, you can do even more for them. As Dr. Paffenberger surmises you will double your time to spend with those other people you are dedicated to. So, what's your logic in not working out now?

The real issue is simpler yet. Again according to the NSGA survey 57% of "couch potatoes" actually want to do more. So, it isn't a matter of "knowing" that inhibits just getting it done. It is a matter of "doing."

Yoda, of Star Wars fame, says it perfectly, "There is no try. Do, or not do." If you are actually in the 43% of sedentary people who don't want to do more, then don't. Keep reading for entertainment sake and make fun of all of us sweating and/or freezing our asses off as we head outdoors for our run. For the rest of you, now just get up and get your ass out the door!

Environment and Geographical Related Excuses

Living in Arizona I could easily make excuses that it is too hot. In the summer, daytime temperatures get as high as 120F and the nights cool down to a mere 90F. I have learned to change my workouts to early in the morning or later in the evening. My workouts consist of running-specific speed-strength workouts that are short but still great quality. When the weather starts to turn cooler, I breathe a sigh of relief and keep running. The flip side is running during the winter in Minnesota. You plan for wind chill factors and wear layers of clothes. In either case, get over it, or run indoors on a treadmill. But, please stop the whining.

Coach, I didn't run because...

93. It's too hot.

94. It's too cold.

95. It's too windy.

96. It's too wet.

97. It's too dry.

98. It's too dark.

99. It's too sunny out.

100. It's too muddy in this desert.

101. The wind was blowing too hard to run.

102. Of a water shortage... don't want to have to take more showers than necessary.

103. The roads are wet.

104. There's no tail wind in my lane.

105. I can't run in the mud.

106. It's a poor track or course.

107. The footing is too soft.

108. The footing is too hard.

109. It's too warm.

110. My glasses fogged.

111. I live in Tucson.

112. I live in Maryland.

113. I live in California. (You get the idea… I'm not going through 50 states and seven continents; insert any place you want.)

114. I'm not alive.

115. I'm from Morocco.

116. I'm from another planet.

117. Nobody runs from where I come from.

118. Nobody runs where I'm going.

119. It's too far to drive.

120. The snake scared me off the trail!

121. I'm afraid to be chased by bulls

122. I'm afraid of the mean mother duck protecting the canal. She attacked me once and almost won.

123. It's too far to drive.

124. It's too far to walk from parking lot to trailhead.

Survey Says... "I've Tried and Failed in the Past"

It is very easy to use what has happened in the past and figure that will happen in the future. It is also human nature to look for and find things to support your theory. You perpetuate and reinforce detrimental beliefs. It keeps you stuck.

Everyone loves success: athletes, coaches, parents, athletic directors, schools, fans. Everyone loves to win or be a winner. And everyone wants to be successful at everything we try. For a surprising number of people, they use this very angle as an excuse not to try in the first place. They make it an excuse. Do you try something actually intending to fail? Not likely. This brings me to my point. If we define ourselves by our victories alone; conversely if we define ourselves by the times we've failed to accomplish what we intended; if we only measure ourselves by "successes" and "failures" then we are certain to completely fail.

First, someone sold most of us a bill of goods that include these themes: "there is only room at the top for one"; "winning is the only thing"; "second place is the first loser"; "all those runners in front of me are more talented"; "I have to accomplish every goal I set"; "if I can't be the best then I won't do it at all"; and "if I don't achieve everything I set out to do – I'm a failure."

I'm as competitive as anyone... just ask teammates, family and friends. I want to do well. I want to "win". But, my wins and losses do not define me.

Excuse Buster

I've participated in 23 marathons (modest by some standards) and I have DNF'd (Did Not Finish) three times. I learned that sometimes, it's Ok just to pack it in. It's not your day. And, contrary to some

belief systems - it is Ok to stop - and come back to fight another day. I've been injured many times only having to fight from the depths of the sedentary world back to athlete.

So, work hard and find joy in the process. I won't tell you to enjoy the pitfalls of being an athlete. Injuries, missed PRs, DNFs, missed Boston Qualifiers, missed age group wins and even breaking a streak of workout days or missing a scheduled workout are all disappointing. I hope in the process, you find that you have developed more character.

So -"failure" – since when were you sold a bill of goods that life was a success-only venture? Change how you view not reaching a goal and then get over it. Just stop using your failures or disappointments as an excuse not to get out and do it. Get your ass up and moving! If your ass sits down again – get someone to kick it!

Personal and Physical Related Excuses

Sometimes physical excuses will prevent an athlete from running. But there are other options to keep the conditioning up. Elliptical, swimming and weight training are just a few of the options available to the athlete that won't allow an excuse to stop them.

Injuries. Sometimes it seems like we are plagued with them. Unavoidable? Sure, just don't do anything. We are engaged in more than merely running, biking and swimming. We do it for more than just "fitness". For most of us, it is an expression of our desire to extend our limits. To go where we think we could go but did not know until we tried. The alternative is not to try, not to endeavor to extend our boundaries. If you think about it, the only way you truly know your limits, is to go beyond them. Then, and only then, do you know what your limits are. Those limits, of course, are for a moment in time. It is a moving target.

Limits change with conditioning (mental and physical) learning and preparation or lack thereof. If you accomplish something it proves that it was within your limits. Whether that something is going faster, further or achieving a promotion at work, in fact, you achieve only what you are capable of. How hard it was to achieve is irrelevant. If you did it, then it was within your capabilities. Again, only by going beyond that and failing or getting injured or dropping out of a race do you learn what you are truly capable of. There is no such thing in human endeavor as greater than 100%. 100% is everything. Math taught us that. You can only give what you got. If you somehow give more, then you were never giving ALL that you had in the first place. You, in fact, were giving less than 100%.

So, to my point, though we never want to encourage injuries and failures, we do want to test limits. When we are injured or we fail at something, it is easy to feel down. It is easy to say, "why am I doing this" or "why try" or "I give up" or "why me". The fact is, we should celebrate something that so many others cannot relate to: our injuries, failures, and "did not finishes" (DNFs) are cause for a celebration of effort. You put it on the line. You tested your limits. I suggest, we celebrate and prepare ourselves both mind and body to do it all over again... even better next time.

In retrospect, I have had many opportunities to celebrate and wouldn't have it any other way. How about you? By the way, you also do have a choice if you never want any more injuries, or never fail or never drop out: just don't do anything. Your couch beckons for your company. For me, I'm coming back! I'm always coming back!

While injured, one of my runners once told me she printed out my statement "I'm always coming back." She put it on her computer monitor. It was her reminder every day that she too would be coming back. I couldn't be happier.

Coach, I didn't run because...

125. I'm a wimp.
126. I have a hole in my heel
127. I feel fat.
128. I'm constipated.
129. I have diarrhea.
130. I'm sore
131. I'm tired
132. I'm grumpy (or grumpier for some)
133. I'm happy
134. I'm moody
135. I'm depressed.
136. I'm recovering from Bloody Nipple Syndrome (BNS).
137. PMS... And if you push me on this you'll regret it!
138. I have angina pain.

139. I'm too sleepy.

140. My heart rate is too high.

141. My heart rate is too low.

142. I don't have a heart rate.

143. I'm not really a runner.

144. I'm not really an athlete.

145. My body fat is too low.

146. My hair hurts.

147. I only had (insert number) hours sleep.

148. The friction from my thighs rubbing together causes too much drag and chafing.

149. I have too much phlegm.

150. I can't get out of bed in the morning and it's too late after school.

151. I can't leave the house because I'm potty training.

152. John broke both my legs.

153. I got Pink Eye (both eyes) and the wind hurts to run, can't close my eyes to run, risk greater injury.

154. I need another day of muscle building (i.e. rest).

155. I have plantar fasciitis

156. I get dizzy going around the track so many times.

157. I forgot.

158. Eye trouble... I couldn't see running today.

159. I have temporary amnesia... I forgot I was a runner.

160. The fire danger is extremely high and I do not feel like shaving my legs.

161. I've had six knee surgeries and now on to other body parts.

162. I'm too old and haven't learned enough to know better.

163. I'm too young and know better.

164. I have no more toe nails.
165. It hurts.
166. I stubbed my toe.
167. I broke my toe surfing.
168. I fell off the treadmill and broke my arm.
169. I fell off the treadmill and broke my nose this time.
170. I fractured my foot and I'm in a walking boot but I can't figure out how to run with the boot on!
171. I injured my pancreas by inhaling little bitty bug larva that was tainted with DDT.
172. I ran out of Body Glide.
173. I suck.
174. I can't stay on my feet.
175. My fat burn heart rate is too low for running.
176. I'm worried about a girl/guy.
177. I'm worried about money.
178. I'm worried about studies.
179. I didn't think.
180. I thought too much.
181. I have shin splints.
182. I have blisters.
183. I have a sore knee.
184. I have a headache.
185. I was snow-blinded.
186. I have cold feet.
187. I thought I was having a heart attack.
188. Too many people are depending on me.
189. No one cared about my performance.
190. I don't like organized athletics.

191. I only run for exercise.

192. I only run for fun.

193. I didn't feel like running.

194. I felt great and that's a bad sign.

195. I couldn't get excited about the race.

196. I was over anxious.

197. My mind was too tense.

198. My mind was too relaxed.

199. I don't like my teammates.

200. My teammates don't like me.

201. I like my teammates TOO much.

202. I got discouraged when _(insert name)_ passed me.

203. I'm looking forward to indoor track.

204. I'm looking forward to outdoor track.

205. I'm not looking forward to anything.

206. I slipped at the start.

207. I can't stand too much stress.

208. I can't stand too much failure.

209. I can't stand too much success.

210. I have emotional problems.

211. I have a bad cold.

212. I can't run anything over a 220 (200).

213. I don't have the courage.

214. I'm chicken.

215. I have to wash my hair.

216. I have Atrial fibrillation with right bundle block.

217. I had a heart attack and they sent me to the cardiac catheterization lab.

218. I have brain cancer and had to go get radiation therapy.

Survey Says…"I'm Too Old to Start"

You don't even want to start on this losing argument. The age 41 record for a mile run is 3:58.13 (Eamon Coughlin). By the way, that was done on an indoor track which is far slower than outdoor tracks. The age 40 5000 (5K) record is 13:43.15 (Mohammed Ezzher). Bob Matteson ran 42.1 seconds for 200 meters; that's the 90-94 year old age group record! Jeanne Daprano ran a 6:47.75 mile to break the world age group record – she's 70 years young. 41 year old Dara Torres, a mom, won three silver medals in the 2008 Olympics in swimming. She did that in a sport thought to be for athletes in their teens and twenties – and that you were far beyond your prime in your thirties. Recently I officiated a track and field meet in which an 88 year old gentleman did the hammer throw, weight throw, shot put and discus. My parents are in their 80s and walk 1-2 miles every morning. If there is inclement weather they walk in the mall. The examples of people of every age getting out and just doing it are too numerous to list here. Go back and read the "investment of time" comments earlier. Then stop lying to yourself and get your ass out there!

Excuse Buster

If there was truly an age limit, you wouldn't see people older than 29 ever doing anything. You wouldn't see people starting to run marathons at age 50. The adage "you are only as old as you feel" is true. But the way you feel younger is to do something not just sit there. Feeling younger is not magic. Feeling younger is not some genetic miracle for a select few. Feeling younger is not from cosmetic surgery. Feeling younger is not in a magic elixir. Feeling young is not from a fountain of youth. Feeling younger is in your hands not someone else's. If time is short, make yourself some time. If you don't want more time because life sucks then just sit there. At least be honest about it and stop the excuses. Otherwise, get your ass up! Get it out the door!

Yet More Excuses

In case the prior 218 excuses weren't enough for you to find a reason to sit home and be a couch potato, there are yet more. But hopefully you're getting the hint that it is just your mindset and it's time for you to just get your ass out the door.

Coach, I didn't run because...

219. Dean won't let me because my club payment is past due

220. It's good recovery... really!

221. There's this one dog...

222. It interferes with my smoking goals.

223. My doctor told me sweating was bad for me.

224. Everybody else isn't doing it.

225. Too much whine.

226. Coach said hard-easy days are good for me... this is my easy day.

227. I don't want to hold everyone up.

228. My puppies trip me.

229. The kitties won't let me run.

230. The dog quit because it was too hot and I had to take him home.

231. My times vary too wildly.

232. I took six years off to be a drag racer.

233. I didn't want to!

234. Sisters rule, and I'm a bro.

235. Coach Dean said so.

236. I missed yesterday so the week is shot now!

237. It was in my horoscope.

238. My physical therapist told me not to run during the summer because the heat will melt the glue in my orthotics.

239. I don't like running.

240. I don't know whether I should warm down or cool down.

241. I can't workout because my neighbor's cat ate my running partner. (With newspaper headlines: "Marathon Mice can run farther, longer")

242. I'm a college student so my alarm clock doesn't have a 5:00AM.

243. I have no one to run with.

244. Yeah, I've been meaning to talk to you about that.

245. What's the point of it?

246. Just DON'T do it!

247. I don't make any excuses.

248. My coach won't let me run. (Coach Dean's fault)

249. My girlfriend/boyfriend won't let me run.

250. I'm running with Tiffany today. (Insert any name you like on this one.)

251. I'm saving myself for ___(insert name of person or event).

252. The bus was too crowded and I couldn't relax.

253. The car was too crowded and I got cramped.

254. The bus is too quiet.

255. I started my kick too soon.

256. I started my kick too late.

257. I can't kick.

258. When I saw that (insert name) was running I choked.

259. I'm a poor starter.
260. The finish judges are poor.
261. I thought there was another lap to go.
262. I ran an extra lap.
263. No medals were awarded.
264. Medals are too cheap to work for.
265. My coach doesn't understand me.
266. I want to reduce my carbon footprint.
267. My doctor told me not to run, said it was bad for my heart.
268. I ran out of EPO and my doctor got arrested.
269. My mother told me not to run.

Survey says… "I Just Don't Want To"

Ok, I added this one. It never shows up on a survey list. But it is probably the most honest answer. It did in fact show up as excuse #233. If you don't want to work out then don't. There isn't a lot to say about this. I'm not here to sell you on something you already intellectually know and cannot argue against. I'm not here to blow smoke up your skirt. Yet, you may still find this book to be handy since all excuses can be used in multiple settings. Be creative and have fun sitting there.

Excuse Buster

No one can make you want to do something you don't want to. However, the logic and science behind the benefits are indisputable.

It is a myth that running deteriorates joints; in fact, running strengthens them. A recent longitudinal study published in the Archives of Internal Medicine by Eliza F. Chakravarty M.D., an immunologist and rheumatologist at Stanford University School of Medicine, pretty much dispelled that myth. They found less frequent joint problems in the runners compared to the sedentary control group. *The incidence of disabilities in the sedentary group was twice that in the running group!*

Running will not shorten your life, it lengthens it. Jim Fixx, author of the Complete Book of Running and often cited as starting the fitness craze in the US, died of a heart attack at the age of 52. Some critics look at this as an example that running failed him. It did not. He started running at age 35 when he weighed 240 pounds and smoked two packs of cigarettes per day. His family had a history of heart disease. His father had a heart attack at age 35 and died of one at age 42. Jim Fixx lived 10 years beyond his father despite his own personal history of a poor healthy lifestyle and a family history of heart disease. He didn't make excuses. He went out and ran. He refused to let a "family history" excuse, an "I'm overweight" excuse or an "I'm a smoker" excuse, stop him from changing and extending his life.

If you won't change bad habits for yourself, do it for someone you love. Find the motivation through others. Do you really want to cheat them out of time with their mother, father, sibling, grandfather, grandmother, son, daughter or significant other? Here may be a sobering thought: imagine their lives without you in the picture. Imagine their pain. Imagine how they will manage without you. Now, it may not be that you are dead and gone. It, in fact, is the same if you cannot be healthy, vigorous and engaged with them while you're alive. You do not have to die, in order not to be there for them. Think about it. Now, get your ass out and run.

Some Everyday Runners Who Just Go Out and Do It

Where's My Shoes? - Taissir Chouman

As a triathlete for more than four years, I'm no stranger to the equipment needed for my sport. I'm meticulous by nature and it carries over in my training and racing as an athlete. I pack my race equipment the night before races. I don't wait until the last minute. I even plan ahead; I will wear one pair of running shoes, and pack a second pair. I never know which will feel better on race day.

Prepared for a personal record, I traveled to California for a Half Ironman Triathlon.

The course was fast. The weather was perfect. I felt great. I knew it was going to be my day. Even my weakest discipline, the swim, went well. I was out of the water with the pack after the 1.2 miles of water. My transition to the bike was smooth as ever. My planning and attention to detail was paying off.

I've worked hard on my biking. It's something I really enjoy. As always, I excelled on the bike section. The 56 miles flew by and I knew I was doing well in my age group. Pulling into the bike-run transition area my focus shifted to getting out of the transition area and running. I knew I needed to find my rhythm right away.

I dismounted from my bike and had my cycling shoes off. I drop my bike on the rack. Then, I look down. I do a double take. Did I place my bike in the right spot? My mind races; I notice one not so minor detail… I don't see my running shoes. Could someone have taken them?

No, in my rush to get on the road from home to California for the race, I slipped on my sandals instead of wearing my running shoes. Not a big deal I figured since I had the second pair in my race bag. But it was a big deal. I never packed the second pair. Both remained on the kitchen counter where I left them… now 350 miles away at home. Going to get them would add quite a bit to my transition time… not a viable option.

I have to admit, what better excuse for quitting is there? How can I run a half marathon without shoes? It's the perfect excuse. Facing a 13.1 mile run, various options race through my head. The first option was to drop out and that was not an option at all. The second option, running barefoot was quickly discarded. The third option was to run in my cycling shoes; sorry not a viable option either. My next option was to knock off one of the other athletes and abscond with their shoes. Ok, I'm not that desperate. And one last gasp option; borrow shoes, but from whom?

I looked around, searching feet. Aha! There stood my wife on the sidelines cheering me on, urging me to get going until she noticed my panicked look. I looked down at my wife's feet. Luckily, she had worn her running shoes that morning. I hollered to her. "Give me your shoes!" She shook her head in disbelief as she ripped them off and handed them over. I barely hesitated as I squeezed my size 10 feet into a woman's size 7 shoe. This was not going to be pretty. But, I was going to finish this thing.

I ran those 13.1 miles and I felt every step of them. For a month, my feet punished me with my absurd decision to run a half marathon in shoes too small. It is now a funny lesson and a great story. But most of all, it showed me and others, that anyone can persevere. And most importantly, that you can either make excuses work for you or make things work!

Lights On — Chris Dragon

The focus to get me out and doing my workout, to me requires some degree of prioritization. They go hand-in-hand. For instance, if I have a long list of things to do at work, but none of them need to be completed that day I am much more apt to be distracted. I could just work on email. I could choose something to work on, get tired of it and shift to something else. On days where I have a deadline looming, focus is not a problem. I MUST get very specific tasks completed. So my solution on those non-urgent days is to figure out (on my drive in to work) what one or two things I would like to get done that day. It is a prioritization exercise which allows me to just focus on one or two things and typically I can avoid distractions (although not interruptions!) that way.

So when we think about our lives, prioritization must incorporate balance. I have three young children and my job which I must balance my running with. Let's face it, from a priority standpoint: family, work, running is the order. This is why I am an early morning runner. If I wait until after work things are more uncertain. Work can run late or I need to take the kids to basketball practice, etc. There are lots of potential for excuses. Doing early morning runs removes 90% of my distractions BUT it does require dedication and focus; especially on those cold, dark, January mornings.

This is how I do it. When the alarm goes off I do NOT hit the snooze button. I get up and go sit down on the toilet in the water closet. Lights on. Door closed. I know this may seem odd, but since I usually have to use the bathroom right as I get up, not only is this is necessary, but is also impossible to go back to sleep sitting on the toilet in a lit room. I will often sit there for nearly 10 minutes slowly waking up. But there is a comfort in knowing that I am not going back to sleep and the process has begun. This routine is always the same. After that I get dressed, brush teeth, etc. and start thinking about the workout ahead. Eventually I am out the door and jogging. The bottom line is that my brain doesn't consider NOT getting out of bed an option. It is simply something that needs to get done. So I do it. I plod through my routine and am always happier for it. The alternative is feeling regretful all day. That is SOOOOOO much worse.

What If? – Christina Heinle

It wasn't the divorce that was causing the tough days. It was the anxiety and depression that made life so challenging. I went through a fifteen week course on anxiety and depression and was trying to use the various tools to help lift my spirits just a little. One of the tools made me a believer of changing your thoughts and not letting your excuses stop you.

While males who suffer from anxiety and depression will often fear having a heart attack, women fear losing their mind. Many days I would feel like I was on the edge of having a nervous breakdown. One day through email a friend made an off-handed comment about me being crazy. Because I worried about going crazy his comments struck a nerve. He had no idea how his words had hurt me. As I sobbed in my office, I didn't know how I could go to track that night. I felt like crap and didn't feel like going. I felt there was no way I could run. And to make it all worse, that night was a mile time trial. Our time trials are supposed to test our condition and demonstrate improvements made. What if I sucked even more than I usually do? What if I'm last…again? All the 'what if's' of how crappy I am and the reasons not to go run were streaming through my head.

The only thing I could commit to was to show up. I went to the track with the intention of doing the warm up and making my excuses for a poor forthcoming time trial. As I was warming up, I thought about that anxiety and depression course. Just as she did in the course, I switched my "what if" thinking. I posed the situation a little differently with these questions. What if I run my best time? What if I have fun? What if I just run to do my best regardless?

It's so easy to use the negative 'what ifs' and let those snowball. But to be an equal opportunity what if-er, you need to give the positive side 'what ifs' as well. Those positive what ifs paid off. I actually ran a personal record that night in my mile time trial. If I had talked myself out of running or allowed the negative 'what ifs' to continue, I wouldn't have had a new personal record and a great boost to my confidence.

Excuses would have robbed me of trying; cheated me from experiencing something I hadn't experienced before (running that fast); and excuses in the end would have whittled away at my self-confidence.

I Forgot My Asthma Pump — Patricia Murphy

As an infant I was allergic to everything. A switch in laundry detergent, a cat nuzzle, or a room left undusted was enough to swell my eyes shut. I remember, when I was about four, a visit to the doctor for allergy tests. He approached me with a board of pins straight out of Abu Gharib and pressed it onto my little blue-white forearm. When the results came back, the doctor said it would be easier to list in my chart the two things I was not allergic to: plastic, artichokes.

Later I started having wheezing attacks. When I was ten years old I complained to my mother that my chest felt tight and that I could hear myself breathing. My mother saw this as a cheap attempt to convince her to stop smoking. But the doctor confirmed I had asthma, and started me on several medications that are no longer administered to humans due to their extreme side effects. I took Theophylline every day until I was in high school. The drug helped, but some of its negative effects were nausea, increased heart rate, and dizziness. Despite my continued use of this maintenance drug and multiple rescue inhalers, I had several severe asthma attacks that sent me to the hospital. In the ER, doctors immediately gave me adrenaline shots and large doses of Albuterol, which sent my heart rate soaring. I came to associate an elevated heart rate and labored breathing with being very, very sick.

Through adolescence and into adulthood, I maintained my fitness mostly through strength training activities and whatever cardio I could find that did not make me feel like I was out of breath. I bought a lifetime membership to Bally's, and I would run or bike to the gym, lift weights for an hour, then run or bike home. I was what I would call a "jogger," who would run/walk up to 5 miles at a pace of 11-12 minutes a mile. Although this allowed me to keep a general level of fitness, I was never particularly athletic.

Then I made a good friend who was just that: athletic. She had played four years of varsity field hockey at Yale. She had completed the New

York Marathon, a feat that seemed unsurpassable. She ran 35 miles a week, for fun. I really wanted to try to add running to my life, and perhaps to one day run a marathon. I knew I would need help to get serious.

That's when I started running with a wonderfully kind and dedicated Coach who encouraged me to try to run faster. But every time I did, my lungs would wheeze and my heart rate would rise. When that happened, it sent me back to those hospital trips as a little girl: being hooked up to machines, the racing heart, and the struggle for breath. It was very hard to separate the two in my mind: fitness and illness. I would run a hard quarter at the track, get very winded and think "I'm going to die." Literally. I often told Coach that I just couldn't do it.

But after a while, and through great encouragement from Coach, I realized that I was not going to die, and in fact, I was getting stronger. Soon I competed in some road races—a 5K here and a 10K there. I managed to push myself to work harder and to mange my emotional responses to running. I began to see physical exertion as a good thing rather than as a threat. I was able to run faster without panicking. Since 2001 I have competed in 50 races from the 5K distance to Half Ironman. I have done running relay races, Mountain Bike relay races, Splash and Dash competitions, and overnight rides for charity. I have won first in my age group in several events.

While I used to use my asthma as an excuse to run easy, now I use it as an excuse to run hard. Because of the cardiovascular fitness I have gained over the past seven years I have been able to decrease my asthma medications and reduce my susceptibility to illness. I still take two maintenance medications a day and I probably will for the rest of my life. But now that I have learned first-hand the benefits of cardiovascular exercise on lung capacity, I will no longer let my asthma be an excuse for not running.

50k Without Excuses — Rob Nichols

I've always seen myself as just your average every day runner. I wanted to do something special after turning 40. But, I didn't want to run just another marathon. No, it had to be an ultra-marathon: 50 miles. I thought about this goal for two years and started formal training a full year out. This goal was so daunting that the list of possible excuses along the journey to accomplishing it was endless.

No matter how well trained you are with miles and miles under your belt, you must practice, perfect, and then follow your race day plan on race day. The two most critical factors you control are: pacing and hydration-nutrition. You do not control the course, the environment, the weather, the competition, or the race organization. Each produces their own set of excuses if you want them. And in my case, a totally surprising variable was uncontrollable – the race distance! The race was shortened from 50 miles to 50k (31.1 miles) by the race organizers only a couple months before the race. The options to find another 50 miler weren't optimal. They would occur months later and necessitate travel out of state. Though disappointed, I refocused on what I controlled and didn't make an excuse not to run or not to do my best.

It is so easy not to pay attention to nutrition and hydration as a working professional. However, I knew there would be no recovering from an inadequate hydration and nutrition plan on race day. The excuse of not planning or not following a plan wouldn't lessen the pain of it all! So I practiced my plan over the course of almost a year of training. Each long run became an experiment in balancing my hydration and nutrition. I used various nutrition and hydration approaches all along the way then evaluated and re-evaluated the effects (before, during and after runs).

I followed my coaches' plan. If I deviated, I always consulted my coaches and made adjustments with their input. I could not have done this without top-notched, well thought out and a well planned training program. I had to trust the coaches and ignore the "fluffy" advice given so freely in magazines and websites. My training program eliminated the guess work and minimized excuse making.

In order to "get it done," I practiced pacing every day. I remained focused on paces and it gave my runs purpose. I ran my quality runs at the prescribed "fast" paces. Goal runs were kept to 8:45 per mile which by the end of training I could click off in my sleep. My running friends nicknamed me The Metronome because of my ability to pace consistently. My easy runs were kept easy even though I often felt like picking it up. I knew if I over-did my easy days, I would have a convenient excuse for not being able to complete the far more critical quality and goal paced workouts.

Saturday morning, on race day, I was up at 4 AM and I began my hydration plan immediately. I had my two cups of medium strength coffee, an ounce of dark chocolate and three toasted Trader Joe's whole wheat muffins with butter and Trader Joe's jelly. Based on my experiments through my training runs, I knew what worked and I didn't need to change in the eleventh hour Then, I continuously consumed water right up to the start. I guess I could have made the excuse that I wasn't thirsty, but I knew that would not be a wise one.

I stuck to my plan throughout the race. I was so engrossed in the run itself I lost track of pacing. I ran what felt comfortable and I fell into a familiar rhythm. I was on automatic pilot. The plan worked well, my legs never felt depleted. I began to feel a little thirsty in the last lap and felt nauseous in the final mile and a half. At that point though, nothing was going to stop me. After finishing, it would have been easy to just collapse, head home, and hibernate on the couch. Instead, I follow my recovery plan. As a result, I indeed recovered quickly from this effort.

It would have been easy to make excuses; excuses not to do the right training, excuses not to plan, excuses not to follow the plan, excuses not to run because it was not the race I intended, excuses about poor nutrition or hydration. Instead, I did set a personal record in the standard marathon distance by 15 minutes in route and kept going to my 50K. I planned around the things I controlled. I set myself up to eliminate or at least minimize any possible excuses not to succeed.

If you are trying to run longer than you've ever run before, here is my parting advice. Give yourself a long enough lead time to succeed. An inadequate or poorly designed training program is a great excuse to crash and burn on race day. Use your long training runs to figure out everything for the race. Where do you chafe? Which clothes are comfortable? What should you eat? How best do you hydrate? Analyze and learn from each run. Then stick with it on race day and just get it done – no excuses.

Oops, There I go Again! - Stephanie Peabody

Single parenting with two busy kids, working full-time as a software engineer and attempting to be a runner is a tough balance. Then, one day it became an even bigger challenge for me.

It was only a few years ago. But I remember it like it was yesterday. It happened. Something I would never expect - a nighttime home invasion. Though my kids were spared the trauma, I was not. I survived and worked through many emotional issues on my way back to both emotional and physical health. At first it was difficult just getting back to some semblance of normalcy.

Running has been a part of my life for more than 15 years. Running outside however for a very long time was emotionally difficult for me. I needed to find my way past the excuse. I loved running outdoors. I loved the freedom. I no longer felt that freedom. Fear replaced that. But, to run; just to run, was far more important. I longed to feel my energy streaming through me stride after stride. It was time to get running again. My compromise was to run on my treadmill either in the early mornings or after my long days of work. Indoor running is safer, convenient and I can keep an eye on the kiddos without arranging a babysitter. It worked.

One early morning, months after the invasion, I was getting ready to work out and the kids were still asleep, I got a phone call at 6:30. The officer on the other end of the line told me the great news – they had caught him! The officer told me to tune into the 7:00 news as they were going to broadcast his capture. I got on the treadmill to run with a sense of needing to let out my emotions of the great news. I never ever had watched TV during running but this had to be an exception. So, I set up the TV for the very first time so I didn't miss the news of his capture. I flipped on the TV and revved up the treadmill.

I warmed up just fine and didn't pay too much attention to the TV as I settled in a bit to my pace. And just as Coach had put down on my schedule, I was going to do fast 200 meter repeats on the treadmill. It's tricky, but I had done it successfully before. I started my repeats. I sped into my next 200, then it came - the special news bulletin flash. The TV caught my attention. I couldn't believe it as I cocked my head to the side – late breaking news, on the scene – they indeed had just apprehended the guy responsible for a series of home invasions including mine. It was him. They had him!

By the way, did you know at that speed on a treadmill it only takes a split second to lose it?

Just then, the whole world went into slow motion. I miss-stepped and I was now in mid-air; arms spread out grasping thin air; legs out behind me; and the whirring treadmill staring in my face. I don't remember the impact. I know I landed face first. The broken nose and treadmill-sanded abrasions on my face were proof of that. It wasn't pretty.

Score: Treadmill – 1, Stephanie - 0.

Despite the face-plant, I was overwhelmed with a sense of relief. They had him. It was still months of emotional processing for me to move on. But, over time healing took place.

That bout with the treadmill should have been enough to knock sense into most reasonable people. But, who said I was reasonable. The hard part was getting back onto the treadmill. I could have easily made any number of excuses; it's dangerous; it isn't really worth it; I'm just too busy to deal with it all. Outside running was not a viable option. I had to get back on the horse and ride. And that I did.

Running progressed smoothly for months. By now the memories of broken noses and flying through the air had long faded. I was running well and feeling great. My confidence was growing and I was looking forward to racing again. It was about six months after the first incident and I was blissfully running my miles on the treadmill. I was in the zone. As I was ending my workout, I went to step off the moving tread.

No sooner did I do so that awful feeling well up within me. "Oh no, not again… nooooooo!!!" I heard the words in my head.

I fought valiantly, but to no avail. I was flying again. The treadmill whirring away as I reached out to stop yet another face plant. My arm stretched out in front of me. Yes! I saved the face plant. Then, snap. I felt my arm give way.

Treadmill – 2, Stephanie – 0.

I called Coach from the emergency room. I proudly reported no face plant, no broken nose; only one broken arm. After he stopped laughing he asked, "At least you can run with an arm in a cast. So, when are you getting back at it?" He's such an empathetic guy.

The fact is that I did get back at it. I was not going to let the treadmill get the best of me. I've kept this up for the past several years. I now do regular runs both outdoors and on my treadmill. I'm training for a half-marathon. I play soccer and roller derby in addition to my running. I think my treadmill episodes prepared me well for these sports. I refuse to let fear run my life. And I don't let something as minor as face plants and broken bones become excuses for not getting my workouts in.

Improve Diet, Running and Stress by Sticking with It - Duane Slade

It was almost a four year journey but I did it. I had plenty of opportunities for excuses along the way. I admit I even used them a few times. But, in the end I'm proud to say I'm a Boston marathon qualifier and finisher.

I have lost over 40 lbs in the past couple of years and I have to say it has everything to do with what you eat – and not making excuses. I was running for five years before I lost any weight. I ran marathons, 5k's, 10k's, half-marathons, and really any event I could. I logged 30 to 40 miles a week and could not get down below 210 pounds I stepped on the scale one day and saw 222 pounds and I had a marathon in two weeks. I decided on the spot that I needed to do something about it.

I found a sports nutritionist. I stuck to her plan and lost nothing for the first two weeks. I was frustrated, but sometimes life is just that way. I kept telling myself that this has to work and that in order to get faster and qualify for Boston I would have to lose weight. At about the two week mark the weight starting falling off. I lost 22 pounds over the next six weeks and that was very motivating. I then started to get into the 190's which I thought I would never see. Pretty soon I was 198 then 195 then 192. I couldn't believe how good I felt and that I was actually looking at getting into the 180's. I woke up one morning and stepped on the scale and there it was, 189 pounds. This was just 15 weeks after I started eating right. Pretty soon I was 187 then 185 then 181. People started telling me how skinny I was and that felt great. They started to ask me how I stayed in such good shape and they credited all of it to my running. I used to run races and people would say things like, 'good job big guy' or 'way to go big fellow'. They don't say that anymore. The motivation to keep it off is all in the way I feel now. Having that feeling in mind keeps away excuses to stray from my healthy diet.

Sometimes I awake in the morning and I think to myself, I don't want to get out of bed and run! I start rationalizing that I ran hard yesterday and my body needs a break. I think that I will just sleep a little longer. I feel this way especially towards the end of a long training schedule. It is very difficult to stay focused and get my workouts in.

Some of the things I do to stay on target, minimize excuses and make sure I get it done are very simple. If I know that I have been feeling out of focus I will invite someone on a run with me. This makes me feel I have to be there because they are there and it always ends up a better quality workout because we push ourselves. Another thing I do when I am feeling the doldrums is make sure I have a plan with variety. I change up my courses and plan running workouts in places that are cool to run in. Two years ago when I was getting ready to run the St. George Marathon and attempt to qualify for Boston, I went and ran the course two times before the race. Along with five friends, we made a road trip out of it and ran different parts of the course over the weekend. It was a refreshing change and the course knowledge we gained was invaluable. Sometimes I will sit down on a Sunday night and look over my schedule and make a plan on where I am going to run each day. I drive to certain areas and will do my miles on certain courses. This gives me something to look forward to and really helps me stay excited about the week of running. All of these things are great, but the thing that keeps me really motivated to run is the feeling I get while I am doing it. It is one of the greatest gifts God has given us, the natural high!

When I am faced with a tough workout I go through a number of different thoughts. Sometimes I psych myself out and feel a little sick the whole time. But I'll do it anyway. For example, sometimes my coach will give me time trials. I hate time trials. If I know they are coming and I prepare the day before mentally then I do great. If I don't prepare mentally, I don't do well and it's pretty demotivating. So, mental preparation for a tough workout is the key for me. I think about each lap or each mile and how I would like to feel. I think about my body running smoothly and efficiently. I like to visualize crossing each time point a little ahead of what coach had planned. I visualize myself breaking barriers and setting personal records. When I do this I always perform better.

Another thing I do when I know I am going to have a tough workout is eat better starting at least two days in advance. I do my speed workouts on Mondays, so I stop drinking any kind of pop on Friday. If I know that I am going to have a tough workout on Monday, I refrain from the ice cream or homemade poppy seed cake on Sunday night. I notice the difference when I eat well and when I don't. In short, completing a tough workout comes down to preparing for the workout before you ever toe the line. I remove an excuse not to just get out and do it.

I recently went through some very difficult times with my work. One of the companies I owned was going through very difficult issues. Friends, associates, and family were affected by it. It seemed to envelop every aspect of my life. Every day was very stressful for almost two years. I remember looking forward to my runs. This was a time that I could just get out and forget about what was going on or I could take a problem and work through it as I ran. On long runs in particular, I would think beforehand about one of my biggest concerns. Then I would set off for my run and start processing every aspect of the problem. By the end of the run I usually had a solution or a good idea of how to better deal with the situation. Running really helped with stress. Instead of life stress becoming an excuse not to run, it became instrumental in problem solving and life balance.

Three Foolproof Approaches to Just Getting It Done!

The Non-workout Approach

It isn't every day that we want to work out, pursue a particular project or goal. Your goal may indeed be worthy of pursuit. It may be ecologically sound (a way of saying it doesn't have some adverse side effects to accomplishing the goal that will deter you.) However, even the most goal-oriented people have times they just don't ALWAYS want to take the next action on their way to that goal. For runners, it may be getting out the door for that workout.

Everyone knows to run a marathon takes months of training. It requires combinations of quantity of runs as well as quality runs. It's easy to map out the workouts; set the plan; set the road map to your destination. Just as with a trip in your car, it's easier to map it than to actually do it. Sometimes there are vehicle breakdowns. Sometimes you run out of gas or have an accident. Sometimes you need to take a break for biological reasons. In the course of pursuing your destination or goal, you will need to find ways to keep the motivation going.

Day-to-day you know you have to do what's on your schedule. After 37 years of running and more than 53,000 miles, there are still days I struggle to get a workout in. Most often it's not physical. In fact, if it is physical then it MAY be a good idea to listen to your body. However, most often the struggle to work out is mental. A long day at work typically is not physically taxing but emotionally draining from the stress and strain. Who feels like getting it together to work out when you are wiped out? For some of us it's easier than others.

So what's a person to do? Commit to a non-committal process.

Huh?

Yes, a non-committal process. This is how it works. Motivation sometimes has to be broken down…to the ridiculous minuscule level sometimes. This is a mind game.

Let me outline a scenario, the actions and the self-talk you need to exhibit to overcome when you don't want to work out.

You arrive home and it's been one of "those" days. You would much rather plop down and watch TV, soak in the hot tub or take a nap.

- First thing to do is to tell yourself, "I'm not going for a run. I'm just going to get out of my work clothes."

- While changing, since you're not going to remain naked. Tell yourself, "Ok, I'll put on my running shorts and t-shirt. I'm only putting them on because they're comfortable. But, I'm not going for a run. I'm just getting comfortable."

- Barefoot and comfy, walk to the kitchen and get a drink of water. You need to go check your mail and you don't want to stay barefoot so you put your running socks on. Repeat to yourself, "I'm just going out to check the mail. I'm not running. I'm comfortable and just going to check the mail."

- Put on your socks and while you're at it, you need shoes on to go check the mail. Running socks and shorts look stupid with dress shoes or heels so put something comfy on... like, say, your running shoes. Repeat to yourself, "I'm just putting my socks and shoes on to check the mail. I am not going for a run. I am just comfy."

- As you walk outside to the mailbox, take deep breaths. Look around and take in your environment... temperature, breeze, sunlight, kids playing outside, traffic. Get your mail and throw away the two-thirds of it that are advertisements. Keep the bills. Notice how many friends didn't write to you today. Take at least three very deep breaths and slowly exhale. Put the mail inside the house.

- Now, decide to just go out the front door. Stand there for a minute. Tell yourself, "I'm not going to run. But, I'm just going to enjoy being outside."

- Put one foot in front of the other slowly. This is called walking. Tell yourself, "I'm not running. I am just moving my body outside. I can go back home anytime I want."

- After a block or so, try moving slightly quicker while telling yourself, "It's not a workout. I'm just moving my body outside. I can go home anytime I want. Some would call this jogging, but I'm just moving forward easily. And, I can stop anytime…"

- Remember, you're not doing a workout. Now, decide to keep moving just one mile. After one mile you decide if you want to continue. You can turn back anytime AFTER that mile now.

A funny thing happens. After a mile of the Non-Workout. Your body begins to flow. The stress of the day melts away. You are in your element once again. Even if it doesn't feel good, you got out. You moved. It is amazing how more often than not it comes together, piece-by-piece, bit-by-bit, step-by-step… closer to your goal.

Try the Non-Workout approach next time you're caught low on motivation.

The Just One More Approach

On days at the track, when I know it will be a challenging workout, my common refrain is "just take it one at a time" or "just focus on this one." Soon after announcing difficult repetitions on the track I often see fear and dread from the runner. At that time I will stress the "just one more" approach.

One day one woman said to me, "You sure say that a lot." Then the other woman chimed in, "Ya, but it really works! I don't want to think about how many of these we have to do. Next thing you know, we're done."

Why does the "just one more" focus work?

1. It chops a large project into bite sized pieces (just like the "eating an elephant" approach). Therefore, psychologically it is less daunting. We think of it as manageable. We can do this. It sets the stage, the mindset, to succeed.

2. It produces a process focus. You can only run one repetition at a time, only do one lap at a time and only run one stride at a time. You cannot do more. Therefore, our mental focus is only on what is most immediately relevant in accomplishing your workout.

3. It focuses on what you control instead of what you don't control. You control your mind, you chose your attitude, and finally you and only you control taking – one more stride, one more lap, or one more "rep".

4. It avoids an outcome focus. We aren't thinking about our final split time totals; or about having completed a certain number of quality miles this week; or about tomorrow's workout; or how sore we will be tomorrow.

5.   **It keeps us in a present focus. We do not control whether we hit our split times on the last "rep." Right now, we do not control if we will hit the next "rep" on time. We only control right now; our current effort; our current determination to maintain pace on the current "rep."**

6.   **It trains your mind! You are practicing the very focusing skills you must have to perform at your best in competition. You will not magically find out how to "focus" to get through bad patches in the middle of a race. You will not magically figure out what to concentrate on in the last miles of your marathon. You must practice the way you race.**

Even if you aren't on the track, this approach works on the roads and trails too! It's just one more step; just one more telephone pole, just one more turn, just one more hill. And in the gym, it's just one more exercise machine or circuit workout station and one more rep.

oach

Focus is a critically overlooked aspect in excuse making. What you focus on is what you get. Focus on how not to get something done, you'll think of a thousand excuses. Focus on how many barriers there are to doing something, the list will be endless.

We lose focus easily. We start off with good intentions. With all the distractions available to us – friends, relatives, TV, Internet, text messages, traffic – it's easy to see how we lose our focus on getting our workouts done.

Focus isn't a single thing. There are actually four "types" of focus within two dimensions identified by sport psychologist Robert Nideffer Ph.D.

The first dimension *breadth of attention* is based on how broad or narrow your attention is focused. The second dimension is *internal and external focus*. This refers to whether you focus on internal feelings and images ("I'm afraid", self-talk) or external stimuli (environment, competition, fans).

When you combine these two dimensions you have four quadrants of focus. All are essential.

A *broad-internal* focus is used to analyze and solve problems, make decisions and develop goals. Example: I'm traveling with a variable work schedule. How do I get my workouts in?

A *broad-external* focus is used to assess what is going on in your environment. Example: Check out that you have your running shoes with you.

A *narrow-internal* focus is used to organize information and mentally rehearse what you will do. Example: Visualize your workouts for the day or week. See the steps you will take to get it done.

A *narrow-external* focus is used to perform or react – actually doing it! This is the focus that is essential to overcoming excuses. Example: Tie my shoes and walk out the door. Run now!

Focus on time you don't have (broad-external) and that will consume you. Focus on where you can squeeze in your workout and you will. Focus on your worries, stresses (broad-internal) and ailments and you will easily find an excuse not to work out. Visualize all the barriers to getting your run in (narrow-internal) and you'll recreate this entire book of lists. If you focus solely on getting out the door and getting it done (narrow-external) you might forget your running shoes.

We routinely alternate between the four. That is not only normal but necessary. A different type of focus is needed for each activity (even aspect of a single activity) we engage in. What gets us in trouble is when we get stuck in one focus or we end up in the wrong focus at the wrong time.

First – you have to establish a workout focus. What is the purpose of your workout today? What pace should you run? How far are you supposed to run? What part of the run do you need to work on (such as hills or late miles when fatigued)? Without a workout focus, your mind will wander. You invite distractions in lieu of an intended focus.

Another step in getting focused is to establish a pre-performance routine to set the stage to get that workout in. This is not only what every elite athlete does. It is what everyday athletes do. You see it with basketball players at the free-throw line. You see it with baseball players getting up to bat. Create your own pattern of actions that lead you to get your workout done just as you read in the story "Lights On" from Chris Dragon. It can include laying out clothing ahead of time; putting shoes on in a certain order; or taking fluids, walking around and doing a specific sequence of stretches. Or mimic Duane Slade who visualizes his workouts before doing them, especially the hard ones. The key is to make it a pattern. The key is to make it predictable. The key is to make it lead to your workout. The key is to reinforce a sequence of actions that lead you to do what you need to do. The key is to get your brain – your mindset – focused on the one thing that needs to get done right now – getting your workout done.

Stop being a victim of circumstances. Stop taking every convenient or popular excuse not to do something. Get your ass out there and run!

Conclusion

If you have read through the excuses you have found some head-scratchers as well as some eye-openers. There are many, what we might call "legitimate", excuses listed. It is most certainly ill-advised to run with a stress fracture for instance. If you read the list to the end you also see an even more serious side to the list. Look back at the list:

#216 Atrial fibrillation; #217 heart attack; #218 brain cancer

Now let me share with you "the rest of the story" about each those situations. Each of these is very real, very sad, and very true.

#216 – I have Atrial fibrillation with right bundle block. His spirit didn't waver; he got treated then he got back running. He just did it.

#217 – I had a heart attack and they sent me to the cardiac catheterization lab. She was back running only weeks after the heart attack and after the stents were inserted into her coronary arteries. Amazingly, she raced a 5K only ten weeks later in 23:07. She just did it

#218 - I have brain cancer and had to go get radiation therapy. She made many of those track workouts… sometimes just the day after her radiation or chemo-therapy treatments; sometimes only able to do a few laps; sometimes not much faster than a fast walk. She just did it. She succumbed to cancer in August 2008, but she never gave up and never made excuses.

THEY are the ones who put these "excuses" on the list, not me. Now, you see how I don't put much stalk in "there isn't enough time." To the individuals with excuses #216, #217, and #218 in particular - time is something precious. Isn't it interesting that they can find some motivation, even humor given the context of the excuses on this list to add their own "excuse?" It is these people who see the folly of everything becoming an excuse NOT to do something. It is these people who lead the way. They struggle like everyone else and more so, but they do it. It is these people I take my hat off to. And they aren't just a number to

Coach Dean

me - thank you John, Claudia and Karen - you are inspirations to me and too many others. It is to you that I dedicate this book.

So, for today, for right now, I say to you - YES YOU - what is your motivation? What are your priorities? Where is your focus? How important is it to get in shape, lose weight or get ready for that next race? Go beyond just thinking about it, go do it. Just for today, regardless of how busy you are, tired you are and limited your time - commit to getting out and doing your workout… just for today… just this once… MAKE the time. Be your own excuse buster.

Now It's Your Turn

You can be a participant in the next edition of "Coach, I didn't' run because..." Submit your interesting excuses or your story of an "every day athlete" who is great at excuse busting to **Excuses@RxRunning. com**.

Do you want to become an Excuse Buster?

Would you like to learn about improving your focus for workouts and racing? If you're interested in a free e-book on how to improve your ability to focus, email your request to **Coach@RxRunning.com.**

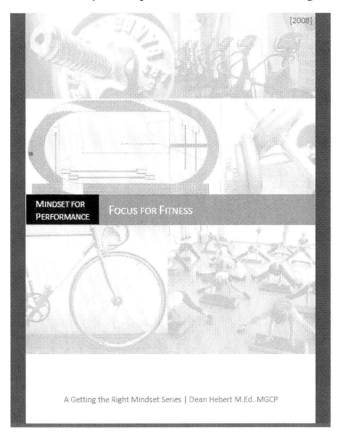

And finally, if you're ready for pushing yourself to the next level and want to overcome some of your own excuses, I can help. It's up to you to take the first step. If you're interested in learning even more about pushing past your excuses, reaching a new level of performance, and want to learn about mental game coaching services I provide, email me at Coach@RxRunning.com.

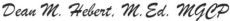

Dean M. Hebert, M. Ed. MGCP

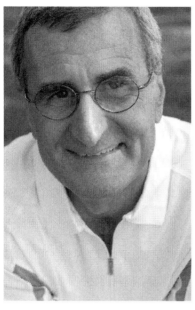

Dean has more than 20 years of coaching, college teaching and workforce training and experience. He has been an invited presenter at many regional and national conferences. He has presented for many professional and non-profit organizations as diverse as MENSA, Body Positive, the Association for Chronic Pain Sufferers, the Western Association of Student Employment Administrators, Head Start, and the American Society for Training and Development. He has won national recognition awards for excellence and a congressional award for service to youth.

After receiving his master's degree, he completed post-graduate work and advanced certification in Sports Psychology. As a certified mental games coaching professional he works with athletes and people in the work place to get the "right mindset."

You have to walk (or run) the talk... and Dean Hebert does! He was named 1996 Masters (over 40) Runner of the Year for the State of Arizona. He set the Arizona 40-45 year old age group 5K record, 15:59.6. With more than 100 career race victories and numerous course records to his name he is a premier state and regional athlete and nationally ranked master's runner. More than 95% of the athletes he coaches have reached new personal records... once they stopped making excuses.

Dean's passion for training is evident in every session he conducts. His style, personality and diverse knowledge-base maintain your attention and offer unique perspectives. Contact him to see, hear and feel the difference he can make to your work team, sports team or organization.

His presentations can become fund raising opportunities for your team or non-profit organization. Ask how!

Mindset for Performance LLC

dba RxRunning & Racing Team

1036 East Knight Lane

Tempe, Arizona 85284

www.RxRunning.com

www.mindsetforperformance.com

http://coachdeanhebert.wordpress.com/

dhebert@mindsetforperformance.com

Coach@RxRunning.com

Printed in Great Britain
by Amazon

52021592R00052